MedicalCenter.com

The Key Facts on Obesity

Everything You Need to Know About Obesity

-Usable Medical Information for the Patient-

By Patrick W. Nee

www.MedicalCenter.com

Published by:

MedicalCenter.com

96 Walter Street/ Suite 200

Boston, MA 02131, USA

Tel: 617-354-7722

www.MedicalCenter.com

manager@medicalcenter.com

Table of Contents

Chapter 1: Introduction

Millions of Americans and people worldwide are overweight or obese. Being overweight or obese puts you at risk for many health problems. The more body fat that you have and the more you weigh, the more likely you are to develop:

- Coronary heart disease
- High blood pressure
- Type 2 diabetes
- Gallstones
- Breathing problems
- Certain cancers

Your weight is the result of many factors. These factors include environment, family history and genetics, metabolism (the way your body changes food and oxygen into energy), behavior or habits, and more.

You can't change some factors, such as family history. However, you can change other factors, such as your lifestyle habits.

For example, follow a healthy eating plan and keep your calorie needs in mind. Be physically active and try to limit the amount of time that you're inactive.

Weight-loss medicines and surgery also are options for some people if lifestyle changes aren't enough.

Reaching and staying at a healthy weight is a long-term challenge for people who are overweight or obese. But it also is a chance to lower your risk for other serious health problems. With the right treatment and motivation, it's possible to lose weight and lower your long-term disease risk.

Definitions of Obesity and Overweight

Overweight and obesity are both labels for ranges of weight that are greater than what is generally considered healthy for a given height. The terms also identify ranges of weight that have been shown to increase the likelihood of certain diseases and other health problems.

For adults, overweight and obesity ranges are determined by using weight and height to calculate a number called the "body mass index" (BMI). BMI is used because, for most people, it correlates with their amount of body fat.

- An adult who has a BMI between 25 and 29.9 is considered overweight.
- An adult who has a BMI of 30 or higher is considered obese.

See the following table for an example.

Height	Weight Range	BMI	Considered
5' 9"	124 lbs or less	Below 18.5	Underweight
	125 lbs to 168 lbs	18.5 to 24.9	Healthy weight
	169 lbs to 202 lbs	25.0 to 29.9	Overweight
	203 lbs or more	30 or higher	Obese

It is important to remember that although BMI correlates with the amount of body fat, BMI does not directly measure body fat. As a result, some people, such as athletes, may have a BMI that identifies them as overweight even though they do not have excess body fat.

Other methods of estimating body fat and body fat distribution include measurements of skinfold thickness and waist circumference, calculation of waist-to-hip circumference ratios, and techniques such as ultrasound, computed tomography, and magnetic resonance imaging (MRI).

Risk Factors for Health Topics Associated With Obesity

Along with being overweight or obese, the following conditions will put you at greater risk for heart disease and other conditions:

- High blood pressure (hypertension)
- High LDL cholesterol ("bad" cholesterol)
- Low HDL cholesterol ("good" cholesterol)
- High triglycerides
- High blood glucose (sugar)
- Family history of premature heart disease
- Physical inactivity
- Cigarette smoking

For people who are considered obese (BMI greater than or equal to 30) or those who are overweight (BMI of 25 to 29.9) and have two or more risk factors, it is recommended that you lose weight. Even a small weight loss (between 5 and 10 percent of your current weight) will help lower your risk of developing diseases associated with obesity. People who are overweight, do not have a high waist measurement, and have fewer than two risk factors may need to prevent further weight gain rather than lose weight.

Talk to your doctor to see whether you are at an increased risk and whether you should lose weight. Your doctor will evaluate your BMI, waist measurement, and other risk factors for heart disease.

The good news is even a small weight loss (between 5 and 10 percent of your current weight) will help lower your risk of developing those diseases.

Causes of Obesity and Overweight

Taking in more calories than you burn can lead to obesity because the body stores unused calories as fat. Obesity can be caused by:

- Eating more food than your body can use
- Drinking too much alcohol
- Not getting enough exercise

Many obese people who lose large amounts of weight and gain it back think it is their fault. They blame themselves for not having the willpower to keep the weight off. Many people regain more weight than they lost.

Today, we know that biology is a big reason why some people cannot keep the weight off. Some people who live in the same place and eat the same foods become obese, while others do not. Our bodies have a complex system to help keep our weight at a healthy level. In some people, this system does not work normally.

Other factors that affect weight include:

- The way we eat when we are children can affect the way we eat as adults. The way we eat over many years becomes a habit. It affects what we eat, when we eat, and how much we eat.
- We are surrounded by things that make it easy to overeat and hard to stay active:
  - Many people do not have time to plan and make healthy meals.
  - More people today work desk jobs compared to more active jobs in the past.
  - People with less free time have less time to exercise.

The term "eating disorder" means a group of medical conditions that have an unhealthy focus on eating, dieting, losing or gaining weight, and body image. A person may be obese, follow an unhealthy diet, and have an eating disorder all at the same time.

Sometimes, medical problems or treatments cause weight gain, including:

- Underactive thyroid gland (hypothyroidism)
- Medicines such as birth control pills, antidepressants, and antipsychotics

Other things that can cause weight gain are:

- Quitting smoking. Most people who quit smoking gain 4 - 10 pounds in the first 6 months after quitting. Some people gain as much as 25 - 30 pounds.
- Stress, anxiety, feeling sad, or not sleeping well
- For women:
  - Menopause -- women may gain 12-15 pounds during menopause
  - Not losing the weight they gained during pregnancy

Understanding Adult Overweight and Obesity

When we eat more calories than we burn, our bodies store this extra energy as fat. While a few extra pounds may not seem like a big deal, they can increase your chances of having high blood pressure and high blood sugar. These conditions may lead to serious health problems, including heart disease, stroke, type 2 diabetes, and certain cancers.

Today, more than two-thirds of adults in the United States are considered to be overweight or obese. More than one-third of adults have obesity. This fact sheet will help you find out if you may be at risk of developing weight-related health problems. It will also explain how overweight and obesity are treated and give you ideas for improving your health at any weight.

Why do people gain weight?

Our bodies need calories (energy) to keep us alive and active. But to maintain weight we need to balance the energy we take in with the energy we use. When a person eats and drinks more calories than he or she burns, the energy balance tips toward weight gain, overweight, and obesity. The tipping point at which the calories coming in and the calories going out become out of balance and lead to weight gain may differ from one person to another.

What other factors are involved?

- Family

  Research shows that obesity tends to run in families, suggesting that genes may contribute to obesity. Families also share diet and lifestyle habits that may affect weight. However, it is possible to manage your weight even if obesity is common in your family.

- The World Around You

  Where people live, play, and work may also strongly affect their weight. Consider the fact that obesity rates were lower 30 years ago. Since that time, our genetic make-up hasn't changed, but our world has.

  The world around us affects access to healthy foods and places to walk and be active in many ways:
  - Many people drive rather than walk.
  - Living in areas without sidewalks or safe places to exercise may make it tough to be more active.
  - Many people eat out or get takeout instead of cooking, which may lead to eating more calories.
  - Most vending machines do not offer low-calorie, low-fat snacks.

Overweight and obesity affect people in all income ranges. But people who live in low-income areas may face even greater barriers to eating healthy foods and being active than other people. High-calorie processed foods often cost less than healthier options, such as fruits and vegetables. There also may be few safe, free, or low-cost places nearby to be active on a regular basis. These factors may contribute to weight gain.

- Culture

  A person's culture may also affect weight:
    - Some cultures have foods with a lot of fat or sugar, making it hard to manage weight
    - Family events at which people eat large amounts of food many make it tough to control portions

- Sleep

  Research suggests that lack of sleep is linked to overweight and obesity. Recent studies have found that sleeping less may make it harder to lose weight. In these studies, adults who were trying to lose weight and who slept less ate more calories and snacked more.

- Medicine

  Certain drugs may cause weight gain. Steroids and some drugs to treat depression or other mental health problems may make you burn calories more slowly or feel hungry. Be sure your health care provider knows all the medications you are taking (including over-the-counter drugs and dietary supplements). He or she may suggest another medicine that has less effect on weight.

Chapter 2: Diagnoses and Symptoms

How are obesity and overweight diagnosed?

The most common way to determine if a person is overweight or obese is to calculate body mass index (BMI). BMI is an estimate of body fat based on comparing a person's weight to his or her height.

Health care providers also look at BMI, along with information about additional risk factors, to determine a person's risk for developing weight-related diseases. Usually, the higher a person's BMI, the higher the risk of disease.

Assessing Your Weight and Health Risk

Assessment of weight and health risk involves using three key measures:

1. Body mass index (BMI)
2. Waist circumference
3. Risk factors for diseases and conditions associated with obesity

Body Mass Index (BMI)

BMI is a useful measure of overweight and obesity. It is calculated from your height and weight. BMI is an estimate of body fat and a good gauge of your risk for diseases that can occur with more body fat. The higher your BMI, the higher your risk for certain diseases such as heart disease, high blood pressure, type 2 diabetes, gallstones, breathing problems, and certain cancers.

Although BMI can be used for most men and women, it does have some limits:

- It may overestimate body fat in athletes and others who have a muscular build.
- It may underestimate body fat in older persons and others who have lost muscle.

Use the BMI Table to estimate your body fat.

Body Mass Index Table

BMI	19	20	21	22	23	24	25	26	27	28	29	30	31	32	33	34	35	36	37	38	39	40	41	42	43	44	45	46	47	48	49	50	51	52	53	54
	Normal						Overweight					Obese										Extreme Obesity														
Height (inches)													Body Weight (pounds)																							
58	91	96	100	105	110	115	119	124	129	134	138	143	148	153	158	162	167	172	177	181	186	191	196	201	205	210	215	220	224	229	234	239	244	248	253	258
59	94	99	104	109	114	119	124	128	133	138	143	148	153	158	163	168	173	178	183	188	193	198	203	208	212	217	222	227	232	237	242	247	252	257	262	267
60	97	102	107	112	118	123	128	133	138	143	148	153	158	163	168	174	179	184	189	194	199	204	209	215	220	225	230	235	240	245	250	255	261	266	271	276
61	100	106	111	116	122	127	132	137	143	148	153	158	164	169	174	180	185	190	195	201	206	211	217	222	227	232	238	243	248	254	259	264	269	275	280	285
62	104	109	115	120	126	131	136	142	147	153	158	164	169	175	180	186	191	196	202	207	213	218	224	229	235	240	246	251	256	262	267	273	278	284	289	295
63	107	113	118	124	130	135	141	146	152	158	163	169	175	180	186	191	197	203	208	214	220	225	231	237	242	248	254	259	265	270	278	282	287	293	299	304
64	110	116	122	128	134	140	145	151	157	163	169	174	180	186	192	197	204	209	215	221	227	232	238	244	250	256	262	267	273	279	285	291	296	302	308	314
65	114	120	126	132	138	144	150	156	162	168	174	180	186	192	198	204	210	216	222	228	234	240	246	252	258	264	270	276	282	288	294	300	306	312	318	324
66	118	124	130	136	142	148	155	161	167	173	179	186	192	198	204	210	216	223	229	235	241	247	253	260	266	272	278	284	291	297	303	309	315	322	328	334
67	121	127	134	140	146	153	159	166	172	178	185	191	198	204	211	217	223	230	236	242	249	255	261	268	274	280	287	293	299	306	312	319	325	331	338	344
68	125	131	138	144	151	158	164	171	177	184	190	197	203	210	216	223	230	236	243	249	256	262	269	276	282	289	295	302	308	315	322	328	335	341	348	354
69	128	135	142	149	155	162	169	176	182	189	196	203	209	216	223	230	236	243	250	257	263	270	277	284	291	297	304	311	318	324	331	338	345	351	358	365
70	132	139	146	153	160	167	174	181	188	195	202	209	216	222	229	236	243	250	257	264	271	278	285	292	299	306	313	320	327	334	341	348	355	362	369	376
71	136	143	150	157	165	172	179	186	193	200	208	215	222	229	236	243	250	257	265	272	279	286	293	301	308	315	322	329	338	343	351	358	365	372	379	386
72	140	147	154	162	169	177	184	191	199	206	213	221	228	235	242	250	258	265	272	279	287	294	302	309	316	324	331	338	346	353	361	368	375	383	390	397
73	144	151	159	166	174	182	189	197	204	212	219	227	235	242	250	257	265	272	280	288	295	302	310	318	325	333	340	348	355	363	371	378	386	393	401	408
74	148	155	163	171	179	186	194	202	210	218	225	233	241	249	256	264	272	280	287	295	303	311	319	326	334	342	350	358	365	373	381	389	396	404	412	420
75	152	160	168	176	184	192	200	208	216	224	232	240	248	256	264	272	279	287	295	303	311	319	327	335	343	351	359	367	375	383	391	399	407	415	423	431
76	156	164	172	180	189	197	205	213	221	230	238	246	254	263	271	279	287	295	304	312	320	328	336	344	353	361	369	377	385	394	402	410	418	426	435	443

The BMI score means the following:

Classification	BMI
Underweight	Below 18.5
Normal	18.5-24.9
Overweight	25.0-29.9
Obesity	30.0 and Above

Waist Circumference

Measuring waist circumference helps screen for possible health risks that come with overweight and obesity. If most of your fat is around your waist rather than at your hips, you're at a higher risk for heart disease and type 2 diabetes. This risk goes up with a waist size that is greater than 35 inches for women or greater than 40 inches for men. To correctly measure your waist, stand and place a tape measure around your middle, just above your hipbones. Measure your waist just after you breathe out.

The following table provides you with an idea of whether your BMI combined with your waist circumference increases your risk for developing obesity-associated diseases or conditions.

Classification of Overweight and Obesity by BMI, Waist Circumference, and Associated Disease Risks

Classification	BMI (kg/m²)	Obesity Class	Men 102 cm (40 in) or less Women 88 cm (35 in) or less*	Men > 102 cm (40 in) Women > 88 cm (35 in)
Underweight	< 18.5	-	-	-
Normal	18.5-24.9	-	-	-
Overweight	25.0-29.9	-	Increased	High
Obesity	30.0-34.9	I	High	Very High

Obesity II	35.0-39.9	II	Very High	Very High
Extreme Obesity	40.0+	III	Extremely High	Extremely High

*Disease risk for type 2 diabetes, hypertension, and cardio vascular disease

**Increased waist circumference also can be a marker for increased risk, even in persons of normal weight.

A primary care doctor (or pediatrician for children and teens) will assess your BMI, waist measurement, and overall health risk. If you're overweight or obese, or if you have a large waist size, your doctor should explain the health risks and find out whether you're interested and willing to lose weight.

If you are, you and your doctor can work together to create a treatment plan. The plan may include weight-loss goals and treatment options that are realistic for you.

Your doctor may send you to other health care specialists if you need expert care. These specialists may include:

- An endocrinologist if you need to be treated for type 2 diabetes or a hormone problem, such as an underactive thyroid.
- A registered dietitian or nutritionist to work with you on ways to change your eating habits.
- An exercise physiologist or trainer to figure out your level of fitness and show you how to do physical activities suitable for you.

- A bariatric surgeon if weight-loss surgery is an option for you.
- A psychiatrist, psychologist, or clinical social worker to help treat depression or stress.

Chapter 3: Treatment

Successful weight-loss treatments include setting goals and making lifestyle changes, such as eating fewer calories and being physically active. Medicines and weight-loss surgery also are options for some people if lifestyle changes aren't enough.

Set Realistic Goals
Setting realistic weight-loss goals is an important first step to losing weight.

For Adults

- Try to lose 5 to 10 percent of your current weight over 6 months. This will lower your risk for coronary heart disease (CHD) and other conditions.
- The best way to lose weight is slowly. A weight loss of 1 to 2 pounds a week is do-able, safe, and will help you keep off the weight. It also will give you the time to make new, healthy lifestyle changes.
- If you've lost 10 percent of your body weight, have kept it off for 6 months, and are still overweight or obese, you may want to consider further weight loss.

For Children and Teens

- If your child is overweight or at risk for overweight or obesity, the goal is to maintain his or her current weight and to focus on eating healthy and being physically active. This should be part of a family effort to make lifestyle changes.

- If your child is overweight or obese and has a health condition related to overweight or obesity, your doctor may refer you to a pediatric obesity treatment center.

Lifestyle Changes

Lifestyle changes can help you and your family achieve long-term weight-loss success. Example of lifestyle changes include:

- Focusing on balancing energy IN (calories from food and drinks) with energy OUT (physical activity)
- Following a healthy eating plan
- Learning how to adopt healthy lifestyle habits

Over time, these changes will become part of your everyday life.

Calories

Cutting back on calories (energy IN) will help you lose weight. To lose 1 to 2 pounds a week, adults should cut back their calorie intake by 500 to 1,000 calories a day.

- In general, having 1,000 to 1,200 calories a day will help most women lose weight safely.
- In general, having 1,200 to 1,600 calories a day will help most men lose weight safely. This calorie range also is suitable for women who weigh 165 pounds or more or who exercise routinely.

These calorie levels are a guide and may need to be adjusted. If you eat 1,600 calories a day but don't lose weight, then you may want to cut back to 1,200 calories. If you're hungry on either diet, then you may want to add 100 to 200 calories a day.

Very low-calorie diets with fewer than 800 calories a day shouldn't be used unless your doctor is monitoring you.

For overweight children and teens, it's important to slow the rate of weight gain. However, reduced-calorie diets aren't advised unless you talk with a health care provider.

<u>Healthy Eating Plan</u>

A healthy eating plan gives your body the nutrients it needs every day. It has enough calories for good health, but not so many that you gain weight.

A healthy eating plan is low in saturated fat, trans fat, cholesterol, sodium (salt), and added sugar. Following a healthy eating plan will lower your risk for heart disease and other conditions.

Healthy foods include:

- Fat-free and low-fat dairy products, such as low-fat yogurt, cheese, and milk.
- Protein foods, such as lean meat, fish, poultry without skin, beans, and peas.
- Whole-grain foods, such as whole-wheat bread, oatmeal, and brown rice. Other grain foods include pasta, cereal, bagels, bread, tortillas, couscous, and crackers.
- Fruits, which can be fresh, canned, frozen, or dried.
- Vegetables, which can be fresh, canned (without salt), frozen, or dried.

Canola and olive oils, and soft margarines made from these oils, are heart healthy. However, you should use them in small amounts because they're high in calories.

You also can include unsalted nuts, like walnuts and almonds, in your diet as long as you limit the amount you eat (nuts also are high in calories).

Foods to Limit

Foods that are high in saturated and trans fats and cholesterol raise blood cholesterol levels and also might be high in calories. Fats and cholesterol raise your risk for heart disease, so they should be limited.

Saturated fat is found mainly in:

- Fatty cuts of meat, such as ground beef, sausage, and processed meats (for example, bologna, hot dogs, and deli meats)
- Poultry with the skin
- High-fat dairy products like whole-milk cheeses, whole milk, cream, butter, and ice cream
- Lard, coconut, and palm oils, which are found in many processed foods

Trans fat is found mainly in:

- Foods with partially hydrogenated oils, such as many hard margarines and shortening
- Baked products and snack foods, such as crackers, cookies, doughnuts, and breads
- Foods fried in hydrogenated shortening, such as french fries and chicken

Cholesterol mainly is found in:

- Egg yolks
- Organ meats, such as liver
- Shrimp
- Whole milk or whole-milk products, such as butter, cream, and cheese

Limiting foods and drinks with added sugars, like high-fructose corn syrup, is important. Added sugars will give you extra calories without nutrients like vitamins and minerals. Added sugars are found in many desserts, canned fruit packed in syrup, fruit drinks, and nondiet drinks.

Check the list of ingredients on food packages for added sugars like high-fructose corn syrup. Drinks that contain alcohol also will add calories, so it's a good idea to limit your alcohol intake.

Portion Size

A portion is the amount of food that you choose to eat for a meal or snack. It's different from a serving, which is a measured amount of food and is noted on the Nutrition Facts label on food packages.

Anyone who has eaten out lately is likely to notice how big the portions are. In fact, over the past 40 years, portion sizes have grown significantly. These growing portion sizes have changed what we think of as a normal portion.

Cutting back on portion size is a good way to eat fewer calories and balance your energy intake.

Food Weight

Studies have shown that we all tend to eat a constant "weight" of food. Ounce for ounce, our food intake is fairly consistent. Knowing this, you can lose weight if you eat foods that are lower in calories and fat for a given amount of food.

For example, replacing a full-fat food product that weighs 2 ounces with a low-fat product that weighs the same helps you cut back on calories. Another helpful practice is to eat foods that contain a lot of water, such as vegetables, fruits, and soups.

Physical Activity

Being physically active and eating fewer calories will help you lose weight and keep weight off over time. Physical activity also will benefit you in other ways. It will:

- Lower your risk for heart disease, heart attack, diabetes, and cancers (such as breast, uterine, and colon cancers)
- Strengthen your heart and help your lungs work better
- Strengthen your muscles and keep your joints in good condition
- Slow bone loss
- Give you more energy
- Help you relax and better cope with stress
- Allow you to fall asleep more quickly and sleep more soundly
- Give you an enjoyable way to share time with friends and family

The four main types of physical activity are aerobic, muscle-strengthening, bone strengthening, and stretching. You can do physical activity with light, moderate, or vigorous intensity. The level of intensity depends on how hard you have to work to do the activity.

People vary in the amount of physical activity they need to control their weight. Many people can maintain their weight by doing 150 to 300 minutes (2 hours and 30 minutes to 5 hours) of moderate-intensity activity per week, such as brisk walking.

People who want to lose a large amount of weight (more than 5 percent of their body weight) may need to do more than 300 minutes of moderate-intensity activity per week. This also may be true for people who want to keep off weight that they've lost.

You don't have to do the activity all at once. You can break it up into short periods of at least 10 minutes each.

If you have a heart problem or chronic disease, such as heart disease, diabetes, or high blood pressure, talk with your doctor about what types of physical activity are safe for you. You also should talk with your doctor about safe physical activities if you have symptoms such as chest pain or dizziness.

Children should get at least 60 minutes or more of physical activity every day. Most physical activity should be moderate-intensity aerobic activity. Activity should vary and be a good fit for the child's age and physical development.

Many people lead inactive lives and might not be motivated to do more physical activity. When starting a physical activity program, some people may need help and supervision to avoid injury.

If you're obese, or if you haven't been active in the past, start physical activity slowly and build up the intensity a little at a time.

When starting out, one way to be active is to do more everyday activities, such as taking the stairs instead of the elevator and doing household chores and yard work. The next step is to start walking, biking, or swimming at a slow pace, and then build up the amount of time you exercise or the intensity level of the activity.

To lose weight and gain better health, it's important to get moderate-intensity physical activity. Choose activities that you enjoy and that fit into your daily life.

A daily, brisk walk is an easy way to be more active and improve your health. Use a pedometer to count your daily steps and keep track of how much you're walking. Try to increase the number of steps you take each day. Other examples of moderate-intensity physical activity include dancing, gardening, and water aerobics.

For greater health benefits, try to step up your level of activity or the length of time you're active. For example, start walking for 10 to 15 minutes three times a week, and then build up to brisk walking for 60 minutes, 5 days a week.

Behavioral Changes

Changing your behaviors or habits related to food and physical activity is important for losing weight. The first step is to understand which habits lead you to overeat or have an inactive lifestyle. The next step is to change these habits.

Below are some simple tips to help you adopt healthier habits.

Change your surroundings. You might be more likely to overeat when watching TV, when treats are available at work, or when you're with a certain friend. You also might find it hard to motivate yourself to be physically active. However, you can change these habits.

- Instead of watching TV, dance to music in your living room or go for a walk.
- Leave the office break room right after you get a cup of coffee.
- Bring a change of clothes to work. Head straight to an exercise class on the way home from work.
- Put a note on your calendar to remind yourself to take a walk or go to your exercise class.

Keep a record. A record of your food intake and the amount of physical activity that you do each day will help inspire you. You also can keep track of your weight. For example, when the record shows that you've been meeting your physical activity goals, you'll want to keep it up. A record also is an easy way to track how you're doing, especially if you're working with a registered dietitian or nutritionist.

Seek support. Ask for help or encouragement from your friends, family, and health care provider. You can get support in person, through e-mail, or by talking on the phone. You also can join a support group.

Reward success. Reward your success for meeting your weight-loss goals or other achievements with something you would like to do, not with food. Choose rewards that you'll enjoy, such as a movie, music CD, an afternoon off from work, a massage, or personal time.

Weight Loss Medicines

Weight-loss medicines approved by the Food and Drug Administration (FDA) might be an option for some people.

If you're not successful at losing 1 pound a week after 6 months of using lifestyle changes, medicines may help. You should only use medicines as part of a program that includes diet, physical activity, and behavioral changes.

Weight-loss medicines might be suitable for adults who are obese (a BMI of 30 or greater). People who have BMIs of 27 or greater, and who are at risk for heart disease and other health conditions, also may benefit from weight-loss medicines.

Sibutramine (Meridia®)

As of October 2010, the weight-loss medicine sibutramine (Meridia®) was taken off the market in the United States. Research showed that the medicine may raise the risk of heart attack and stroke.

Orlistat (Xenical® and Alli®)

Orlistat (Xenical®) causes a weight loss between 5 and 10 pounds, although some people lose more weight. Most of the weight loss occurs within the first 6 months of taking the medicine.

People taking Xenical need regular checkups with their doctors, especially during the first year of taking the medicine. During checkups, your doctor will check your weight, blood pressure, and pulse and may recommend other tests. He or she also will talk with you about any medicine side effects and answer your questions.

The FDA also has approved Alli®, an over-the-counter (OTC) weight-loss aid for adults. Alli is the lower dose form of orlistat. Alli is meant to be used along with a reduced-calorie, low-fat diet and physical activity. In studies, most people taking Alli lost 5 to 10 pounds over 6 months.

Both Xenical and Alli reduce the absorption of fats, fat calories, and vitamins A, D, E, and K to promote weight loss. Both medicines also can cause mild side effects, such as oily and loose stools.

Although rare, some reports of liver disease have occurred with the use of orlistat. More research is needed to find out whether the medicine plays a role in causing liver disease. Talk with your doctor if you're considering using Xenical or Alli to lose weight. He or she can discuss the risks and benefits with you.

You also should talk with your doctor before starting orlistat if you're taking blood-thinning medicines or being treated for diabetes or thyroid disease. Also, ask your doctor whether you should take a multivitamin due to the possible loss of some vitamins.

Lorcaserin Hydrochloride (Belviq®) and Qsymia™

In July 2012, the FDA approved two new medicines for chronic (ongoing) weight management. Lorcaserin hydrochloride (Belviq®) and Qsymia™ are approved for adults who have a BMI of 30 or greater. (Qsymia is a combination of two FDA-approved medicines: phentermine and topiramate.)

These medicines also are approved for adults with a BMI of 27 or greater who have at least one weight-related condition, such as high blood pressure, type 2 diabetes, or high blood cholesterol.

Both medicines are meant to be used along with a reduced-calorie diet and physical activity.

Other Medicines

Some prescription medicines are used for weight loss, but aren't FDA-approved for treating obesity. They include:

- Medicines to treat depression. Some medicines for depression cause an initial weight loss and then a regain of weight while taking the medicine.
- Medicines to treat seizures. Two medicines used for seizures, topiramate and zonisamide, have been shown to cause weight loss. These medicines are being studied to see whether they will be useful in treating obesity.

- Medicines to treat diabetes. Metformin may cause small amounts of weight loss in people who have obesity and diabetes. It's not known how this medicine causes weight loss, but it has been shown to reduce hunger and food intake.

Over-the-Counter Products

Some OTC products claim to promote weight loss. The FDA doesn't regulate these products because they're considered dietary supplements, not medicines.

However, many of these products have serious side effects and generally aren't recommended. Some of these OTC products include:

- Ephedra (also called ma huang). Ephedra comes from plants and has been sold as a dietary supplement. The active ingredient in the plant is called ephedrine. Ephedra can cause short-term weight loss, but it also has serious side effects. It causes high blood pressure and stresses the heart. In 2004, the FDA banned the sale of dietary supplements containing ephedra in the United States.
- Chromium. This is a mineral that's sold as a dietary supplement to reduce body fat. While studies haven't found any weight-loss benefit from chromium, there are few serious side effects from taking it.
- Diuretics and herbal laxatives. These products cause you to lose water weight, not fat. They also can lower your body's potassium levels, which may cause heart and muscle problems.

- Hoodia. Hoodia is a cactus that's native to Africa. It's sold in pill form as an appetite suppressant. However, no firm evidence shows that hoodia works. No large-scale research has been done on humans to show whether hoodia is effective or safe.

Weight-Loss Surgery

Weight-loss surgery might be an option for people who have extreme obesity (BMI of 40 or more) when other treatments have failed.

Weight-loss surgery also is an option for people who have a BMI of 35 or more and life-threatening conditions, such as:

- Severe sleep apnea (a condition in which you have one or more pauses in breathing or shallow breaths while you sleep)
- Obesity-related cardiomyopathy (KAR-de-o-mi-OP-ah-thee; diseases of the heart muscle)
- Severe type 2 diabetes

Types of Weight-Loss Surgery

Two common weight-loss surgeries include banded gastroplasty and Roux-en-Y gastric bypass. For gastroplasty, a band or staples are used to create a small pouch at the top of your stomach. This surgery limits the amount of food and liquids the stomach can hold.

For gastric bypass, a small stomach pouch is created with a bypass around part of the small intestine where most of the calories you eat are absorbed. This surgery limits food intake and reduces the calories your body absorbs.

Weight-loss surgery can improve your health and weight. However, the surgery can be risky, depending on your overall health. Gastroplasty has few long-term side effects, but you must limit your food intake dramatically.

Gastric bypass has more side effects. They include nausea (feeling sick to your stomach), bloating, diarrhea, and faintness. These side effects are all part of a condition called dumping syndrome. After gastric bypass, you may need multivitamins and minerals to prevent nutrient deficiencies.

Lifelong medical followup is needed after both surgeries. Your doctor also may recommend a program both before and after surgery to help you with diet, physical activity, and coping skills.

If you think you would benefit from weight-loss surgery, talk with your doctor. Ask whether you're a candidate for the surgery and discuss the risks, benefits, and what to expect.

Weight-Loss Maintenance

Maintaining your weight loss over time can be a challenge. For adults, weight loss is a success if you lose at least 10 percent of your initial weight and you don't regain more than 6 or 7 pounds in 2 years. You also must keep a lower waist circumference (at least 2 inches lower than your waist circumference before you lost weight).

After 6 months of keeping off the weight, you can think about losing more if:

- You've already lost 5 to 10 percent of your body weight

- You're still overweight or obese

The key to losing more weight or maintaining your weight loss is to continue with lifestyle changes. Adopt these changes as a new way of life.

If you want to lose more weight, you may need to eat fewer calories and increase your activity level. For example, if you eat 1,600 calories a day but don't lose weight, you may want to cut back to 1,200 calories. It's also important to make physical activity part of your normal daily routine.

Chapter 4: Prevention

Healthy Lifestyles

Following a healthy lifestyle can help you prevent overweight and obesity. Many lifestyle habits begin during childhood. Thus, parents and families should encourage their children to make healthy choices, such as following a healthy diet and being physically active.

Make following a healthy lifestyle a family goal. For example:

- Follow a healthy eating plan. Make healthy food choices, keep your calorie needs and your family's calorie needs in mind, and focus on the balance of energy IN and energy OUT.
- Focus on portion size. Watch the portion sizes in fast food and other restaurants. The portions served often are enough for two or three people. Children's portion sizes should be smaller than those for adults. Cutting back on portion size will help you balance energy IN and energy OUT.
- Be active. Make personal and family time active. Find activities that everyone will enjoy. For example, go for a brisk walk, bike or rollerblade, or train together for a walk or run.
- Reduce screen time. Limit the use of TVs, computers, DVDs, and videogames because they limit time for physical activity. Health experts recommend 2 hours or less a day of screen time that's not work- or homework-related.

- Keep track of your weight, body mass index, and waist circumference. Also, keep track of your children's growth.

Led by the National Heart, Lung, and Blood Institute, four Institutes from the National Institutes of Health have come together to promote *We Can!®—Ways to Enhance Children's Activity & Nutrition.*

We Can! is a national education program designed for parents and caregivers to help children 8 to 13 years old maintain a healthy weight. The evidence-based program offers parents and families tips and fun activities to encourage healthy eating, increase physical activity, and reduce time spent being inactive.

Currently, more than 140 community groups around the country are participating in *We Can!* programs for parents and youth. These community groups include hospitals, health departments, clinics, faith-based organizations, YMCAs, schools, and more.

Energy Balance

Energy is another word for "calories." Your energy balance is the balance of calories consumed through eating and drinking compared to calories burned through physical activity. What you eat and drink is ENERGY IN. What you burn through physical activity is ENERGY OUT.

You burn a certain number of calories just by breathing air and digesting food. You also burn a certain number of calories (ENERGY OUT) through your daily routine. For example, children burn calories just being students—walking to their lockers, carrying books, etc.—and adults burn calories walking to the bus stop, going shopping, etc. A chart of estimated calorie requirements for children and adults is available at the link below; this chart can help you maintain a healthy calorie balance.

An important part of maintaining energy balance is the amount of ENERGY OUT (physical activity) that you do. People who are more physically active burn more calories than those who are not as physically active.

The same amount of ENERGY IN (calories consumed) and ENERGY OUT (calories burned) over time = weight stays the same
More IN than OUT over time = weight gain
More OUT than IN over time = weight loss

Your ENERGY IN and OUT don't have to balance every day. It's having a balance over time that will help you stay at a healthy weight for the long term. Children need to balance their energy, too, but they're also growing and that should be considered as well. Energy balance in children happens when the amount of ENERGY IN and ENERGY OUT supports natural growth without promoting excess weight gain.

That's why you should take a look at the Estimated Calorie Requirement chart, to get a sense of how many calories (ENERGY IN) you and your family need on a daily basis.

Estimated Calorie Requirements
This calorie requirement chart presents estimated amounts of calories needed to maintain energy balance (and a healthy body weight) for various gender and age groups at three

different levels of physical activity. The estimates are rounded to the nearest 200 calories and were determined using an equation from the Institute of Medicine (IOM).

Gender	Age (years)	Activity Level		
		Sedentary	Moderately Active	Active
Child	2-3	1,000	1,000 - 1,400	1,000 - 1,400
Female	4 - 8	1,200	1,400 - 1,600	1,400 - 1,800
Female	9-13	1,600	1,600 - 2,000	1,800 - 2,000
Female	14-18	1,800	2,000	2,400
Female	19-30	2,000	2,000 - 2,200	2,400
Female	31-50	1,800	2,000	2,200
Female	51+	1,600	1,800	2,000 - 2,200
Male	4-8	1,400	1,400 - 1,600	1,600 - 2,000
Male	9-13	1,800	1,800 - 2,200	2,000 - 2,600

Gender	Age (years)	Activity Level		
		Sedentary	Moderately Active	Active
Male	14-18	2,200	2,400 - 2,800	2,800 - 3,200
Male	19-30	2,400	2,600 - 2,800	3,000
Male	31-50	2,200	2,400 - 2,600	2,800 - 3,000
Male	51+	2,000	2,200 - 2,400	2,400 - 2,800

- These levels are based on Estimated Energy Requirements (EER) from the IOM Dietary Reference Intakes macronutrients report, 2002, calculated by gender, age, and activity level for reference-sized individuals. "Reference size," as determined by IOM, is based on median height and weight for ages up to 18 years of age and median height and weight for that height to give a BMI of 21.5 for adult females and 22.5 for adult males.
- Sedentary means a lifestyle that includes only light physical activity associated with typical day-to-day life.
- Moderately active means a lifestyle that includes physical activity equivalent to walking about 1.5 to 3

miles per day at 3 to 4 miles per hour, in addition to the light physical activity associated with typical day-to-day life.

- Active means a lifestyle that includes physical activity equivalent to walking more than 3 miles per day at 3 to 4 miles per hour, in addition to the light physical activity associated with typical day-to-day life.

- The calorie ranges shown are to accommodate needs of different ages within the group. For children and adolescents, more calories are needed at older ages. For adults, fewer calories are needed at older ages.

Energy Balance in Real Life

Think of it as balancing your "lifestyle budget." For example, if you know you and your family will be going to a party and may eat more high-calorie foods than normal, then you may wish to eat fewer calories for a few days before so that it balances out. Or, you can increase your physical activity level for the few days before or after the party, so that you can burn off the extra energy.

The same applies to your kids. If they'll be going to a birthday party and eating cake and ice cream—or other foods high in fat and added sugar—help them balance their calories the day before and/or after by providing ways for them to be more physically active.

Here's another way of looking at energy balance in real life.

Eating just 150 calories more a day than you burn can lead to an extra 5 pounds over 6 months. That's a gain of 10 pounds a year. If you don't want this weight gain to happen, or you want to lose the extra weight, you can either reduce your ENERGY IN or increase your ENERGY OUT. Doing both is the best way to achieve and maintain a healthy body weight.

- Here are some ways to cut 150 calories (ENERGY IN):
    - Drink water instead of a 12-ounce regular soda
    - Order a small serving of French fries instead of a medium , or order a salad with dressing on the side instead
    - Eat an egg-white omelet (with three eggs), instead of whole eggs
    - Use tuna canned in water (6-ounce can), instead of oil
- Here are some ways to burn 150 calories (ENERGY OUT), in just 30 minutes (for a 150 pound person):
    - Shoot hoops
    - Walk two miles
    - Do yard work (gardening, raking leaves, etc.)
    - Go for a bike ride
    - Dance with your family or friends

Chapter 5: Health Risks of Obesity and Overweight

What kinds of health problems are linked to overweight and obesity?

Excess weight may increase the risk for many health problems, including

- type 2 diabetes
- high blood pressure
- heart disease and strokes
- certain types of cancer
- sleep apnea
- osteoarthritis
- fatty liver disease
- kidney disease
- pregnancy problems, such as high blood sugar during pregnancy, high blood pressure, and increased risk for cesarean delivery (C-section)

How can I tell if I weigh too much?

Gaining a few pounds during the year may not seem like a big deal. But these pounds can add up over time.

How can you tell if your weight could increase your chances of developing health problems? Knowing two numbers may help you understand your risk: your body mass index (BMI) score and your waist size in inches.

Body Mass Index

The BMI is one way to tell whether you are at a normal weight, are overweight, or have obesity. It measures your weight in relation to your height and provides a score to help place you in a category:

- normal weight: BMI of 18.5 to 24.9
- overweight: BMI of 25 to 29.9
- obesity: BMI of 30 or higher

Waist Size

Another important number to know is your waist size in inches. Having too much fat around your waist may increase health risks even more than having fat in other parts of your body.

Women with a waist size of more than 35 inches and men with a waist size of more than 40 inches may have higher chances of developing diseases related to obesity.

Know Your Health Numbers

Measure	Target
Target BMI	18.5–24.9
Waist size	Men: less than 40 in. Women: less than 35 in.
Blood pressure	120/80 mm Hg or less
LDL (bad cholesterol)	Less than 100 mg/dL
HDL (good cholesterol)	Men: more than 40 mg/dL Women: more than 50 mg/dL
Triglycerides	Less than 150 mg/dL
Blood sugar (fasting)	Less than 100 mg/dL

How can I lower my risk of having health problems related to overweight and obesity?

If you are considered to be overweight, losing as little as 5 percent of your body weight may lower your risk for several diseases, including heart disease and type 2 diabetes. If you weigh 200 pounds, this means losing 10 pounds. Slow and steady weight loss of 1/2 to 2 pounds per week, and not more than 3 pounds per week, is the safest way to lose weight.

Federal guidelines on physical activity recommend that you get at least 150 minutes a week of moderate aerobic activity (like biking or brisk walking). To lose weight, or to maintain weight loss, you may need to be active for up to 300 minutes per week. You also need to do activities to strengthen muscles (like push-ups or sit-ups) at least twice a week.

Federal dietary guidelines recommend many tips for healthy eating that may also help you control your weight. Here are a few examples:

- Make half of your plate fruits and vegetables.
- Replace unrefined grains (white bread, pasta, white rice) with whole-grain options (whole wheat bread, brown rice, oatmeal).
- Enjoy lean sources of protein, such as lean meats, seafood, beans and peas, soy, nuts, and seeds.

For some people who have obesity and related health problems, bariatric (weight-loss) surgery may be an option. Bariatric surgery has been found to be effective in promoting weight loss and reducing the risk for many health problems.

Type 2 Diabetes

What is type 2 diabetes?

Type 2 diabetes is a disease in which blood sugar levels are above normal. High blood sugar is a major cause of heart disease, kidney disease, stroke, amputation, and blindness. In 2009, diabetes was the seventh leading cause of death in the United States.

Type 2 diabetes is the most common type of diabetes. Family history and genes play a large role in type 2 diabetes. Other risk factors include a low activity level, poor diet, and excess body weight around the waist. In the United States, type 2 diabetes is more common among blacks, Latinos, and American Indians than among whites.

How is type 2 diabetes linked to overweight?

About 80 percent of people with type 2 diabetes are overweight or obese.5 It isn't clear why people who are overweight are more likely to develop this disease. It may be that being overweight causes cells to change, making them resistant to the hormone insulin. Insulin carries sugar from blood to the cells, where it is used for energy. When a person is insulin resistant, blood sugar cannot be taken up by the cells, resulting in high blood sugar. In addition, the cells that produce insulin must work extra hard to try to keep blood sugar normal. This may cause these cells to gradually fail.

How can weight loss help?

If you are at risk for type 2 diabetes, losing weight may help prevent or delay the onset of diabetes. If you have type 2 diabetes, losing weight and becoming more physically active can help you control your blood sugar levels and prevent or delay health problems. Losing weight and exercising more may also allow you to reduce the amount of diabetes medicine you take.

Diabetes Prevention Program

The Diabetes Prevention Program (DPP) was a large clinical study sponsored by the National Institutes of Health to look at ways to prevent type 2 diabetes in adults who were overweight.

The DPP found that losing just 5 to 7 percent of your body weight and doing moderately intense exercise (like brisk walking) for 150 minutes a week may prevent or delay the onset of type 2 diabetes.

High Blood Pressure

What is high blood pressure?

Every time your heart beats, it pumps blood through your arteries to the rest of your body. Blood pressure is how hard your blood pushes against the walls of your arteries. High blood pressure (hypertension) usually has no symptoms, but it may cause serious problems, such as heart disease, stroke, and kidney failure.

A blood pressure of 120/80 mm Hg (often referred to as "120 over 80") is considered normal. If the top number (systolic blood pressure) is consistently 140 or higher or the bottom number (diastolic blood pressure) is 90 or higher, you are considered to have high blood pressure.

How is high blood pressure linked to overweight?

High blood pressure is linked to overweight and obesity in several ways. Having a large body size may increase blood pressure because your heart needs to pump harder to supply blood to all your cells. Excess fat may also damage your kidneys, which help regulate blood pressure.

How can weight loss help?

Weight loss that will get you close to the normal BMI range may greatly lower high blood pressure. Other helpful changes are to quit smoking, reduce salt, and get regular physical activity. However, if lifestyle changes aren't enough, your doctor may prescribe drugs to lower your blood pressure.

Heart Disease

What is heart disease?

Heart disease is a term used to describe several problems that may affect your heart. The most common type of problem happens when a blood vessel that carries blood to the heart becomes hard and narrow. This may keep the heart from getting all the blood it needs. Other problems may affect how well the heart pumps. If you have heart disease, you may suffer from a heart attack, heart failure, sudden cardiac death, angina (chest pain), or abnormal heart rhythm. Heart disease is the leading cause of death in the United States.

How is heart disease linked to overweight?

People who are overweight or obese often have health problems that may increase the risk for heart disease. These health problems include high blood pressure, high cholesterol, and high blood sugar. In addition, excess weight may cause changes to your heart that make it work harder to send blood to all the cells in your body.

How can weight loss help?

Losing 5 to 10 percent of your weight may lower your chances of developing heart disease. If you weigh 200 pounds, this means losing as little as 10 pounds. Weight loss may improve blood pressure, cholesterol levels, and blood flow.

Stroke

What is a stroke?

A stroke happens when the flow of blood to a part of your brain stops, causing brain cells to die. The most common type of stroke, called ischemic stroke, occurs when a blood clot blocks an artery that carries blood to the brain. Another type of stroke, called hemorrhagic stroke, happens when a blood vessel in the brain bursts.

How are strokes linked to overweight?

Overweight and obesity are known to increase blood pressure. High blood pressure is the leading cause of strokes. Excess weight also increases your chances of developing other problems linked to strokes, including high cholesterol, high blood sugar, and heart disease.

How can weight loss help?

One of the most important things you can do to reduce your stroke risk is to keep your blood pressure under control. Losing weight may help you lower your blood pressure. It may also improve your cholesterol and blood sugar, which may then lower your risk for stroke.

Sleep Apnea

What is sleep apnea?

Sleep apnea is a condition in which a person has one or more pauses in breathing during sleep. A person who has sleep apnea may suffer from daytime sleepiness, difficulty focusing, and even heart failure.

How is sleep apnea linked to overweight?

Obesity is the most important risk factor for sleep apnea. A person who is overweight may have more fat stored around his or her neck. This may make the airway smaller. A smaller airway can make breathing difficult or loud (because of snoring), or breathing may stop altogether for short periods of time. In addition, fat stored in the neck and throughout the body may produce substances that cause inflammation. Inflammation in the neck is a risk factor for sleep apnea.

How can weight loss help?

Weight loss usually improves sleep apnea. Weight loss may help to decrease neck size and lessen inflammation.

Osteoarthritis

What is osteoarthritis?

Osteoarthritis is a common health problem that causes pain and stiffness in your joints. Osteoarthritis is often related to aging or to an injury, and most often affects the joints of the hands, knees, hips, and lower back.

How is osteoarthritis linked to overweight?

Being overweight is one of the risk factors for osteoarthritis, along with joint injury, older age, and genetic factors. Extra weight may place extra pressure on joints and cartilage (the hard but slippery tissue that covers the ends of your bones at a joint), causing them to wear away. In addition, people with more body fat may have higher blood levels of substances that cause inflammation. Inflamed joints may raise the risk for osteoarthritis.

How can weight loss help?

For those who are overweight or obese, losing weight may help reduce the risk of developing osteoarthritis. Weight loss of at least 5 percent of your body weight may decrease stress on your knees, hips, and lower back and lessen inflammation in your body.

If you have osteoarthritis, losing weight may help improve your symptoms. Research also shows that exercise is one of the best treatments for osteoarthritis. Exercise can improve mood, decrease pain, and increase flexibility.

Fatty Liver Disease

What is fatty liver disease?

Fatty liver disease, also known as nonalcoholic steatohepatitis (NASH), occurs when fat builds up in the liver and causes injury. Fatty liver disease may lead to severe liver damage, cirrhosis (scar tissue), or even liver failure.

Fatty liver disease usually produces mild or no symptoms. It is like alcoholic liver disease, but it isn't caused by alcohol and can occur in people who drink little or no alcohol.

How is fatty liver disease linked to overweight?

The cause of fatty liver disease is still not known. The disease most often affects people who are middle-aged, overweight or obese, and/or diabetic. Fatty liver disease may also affect children.

How can weight loss help?

Although there is no specific treatment for fatty liver disease, patients are generally advised to lose weight, eat a healthy diet, increase physical activity, and avoid drinking alcohol. If you have fatty liver disease, lowering your body weight to a healthy range may improve liver tests and reverse the disease to some extent.

Kidney Disease

What is kidney disease?

Your kidneys are two bean-shaped organs that filter blood, removing extra water and waste products, which become urine. Your kidneys also help control blood pressure so that your body can stay healthy.

Kidney disease means that the kidneys are damaged and can't filter blood like they should. This damage can cause wastes to build up in the body. It can also cause other problems that can harm your health.

How is kidney disease linked to overweight?

Obesity increases the risk of diabetes and high blood pressure, the most common causes of chronic kidney disease. Recent studies suggest that even in the absence of these risks, obesity itself may promote chronic kidney disease and quicken its progress.

How can weight loss help?

If you are in the early stages of chronic kidney disease, losing weight may slow the disease and keep your kidneys healthier longer. You should also choose foods with less salt (sodium), keep your blood pressure under control, and keep your blood glucose in the target range.

Pregnancy Problems

What are pregnancy problems?

Overweight and obesity raise the risk of health problems for both mother and baby that may occur during pregnancy. Pregnant women who are overweight or obese may have an increased risk for

- developing gestational diabetes (high blood sugar during pregnancy)
- having preeclampsia (high blood pressure during pregnancy that can cause severe problems for both mother and baby if left untreated)
- needing a C-section and, as a result, taking longer to recover after giving birth

Babies of overweight or obese mothers are at an increased risk of being born too soon, being stillborn (dead in the womb after 20 weeks of pregnancy), and having neural tube defects (defects of the brain and spinal cord).

How are pregnancy problems linked to overweight?

Pregnant women who are overweight are more likely to develop insulin resistance, high blood sugar, and high blood pressure. Overweight also increases the risks associated with surgery and anesthesia, and severe obesity increases surgery time and blood loss.

Gaining too much weight during pregnancy can have long-term effects for both mother and child. These effects include that the mother will have overweight or obesity after the child is born. Another risk is that the baby may gain too much weight later as a child or as an adult.

How many pounds should I gain during pregnancy?

Pre-pregnancy Weight	Amount to Gain
Underweight (BMI < 18.5)	28–40 lbs.
Normal Weight (BMI 18.5–24.9)	25–35 lbs.
Overweight (BMI 25–29.9)	15–25 lbs.
Obesity (BMI 30+)	11–20 lbs.

How can weight loss help?

If you are overweight or obese and would like to become pregnant, talk to your health care provider about losing weight first. Reaching a normal weight before becoming pregnant may reduce your chances of developing weight-related problems. Pregnant women who are overweight or obese should speak with their health care provider about limiting weight gain and being physically active during pregnancy.

Losing excess weight after delivery may help women reduce their health risks. For example, if a woman developed gestational diabetes, losing weight may lower her risk of developing diabetes later in life.

Cancer

- During the past several decades, the percentage of overweight and obese adults and children has increased markedly.

- Obesity is associated with increased risks of cancers of the esophagus, breast (postmenopausal), endometrium (the lining of the uterus), colon and rectum, kidney, pancreas, thyroid, gallbladder, and possibly other cancer types.
- Obese people are also at higher risk of coronary heart disease, stroke, high blood pressure, diabetes, and a number of other chronic diseases.

What is known about the relationship between obesity and cancer?

Obesity is associated with increased risks of the following cancer types, and possibly others as well:

- Esophagus
- Pancreas
- Colon and rectum
- Breast (after menopause)
- Endometrium (lining of the uterus)
- Kidney
- Thyroid
- Gallbladder

One study, using NCI Surveillance, Epidemiology, and End Results (SEER) data, estimated that in 2007 in the United States, about 34,000 new cases of cancer in men (4 percent) and 50,500 in women (7 percent) were due to obesity. The percentage of cases attributed to obesity varied widely for different cancer types but was as high as 40 percent for some cancers, particularly endometrial cancer and esophageal adenocarcinoma.

A projection of the future health and economic burden of obesity in 2030 estimated that continuation of existing trends in obesity will lead to about 500,000 additional cases of cancer in the United States by 2030. This analysis also found that if every adult reduced their BMI by 1 percent, which would be equivalent to a weight loss of roughly 1 kg (or 2.2 lbs) for an adult of average weight, this would prevent the increase in the number of cancer cases and actually result in the avoidance of about 100,000 new cases of cancer.

Several possible mechanisms have been suggested to explain the association of obesity with increased risk of certain cancers:

- Fat tissue produces excess amounts of estrogen, high levels of which have been associated with the risk of breast, endometrial, and some other cancers.
- Obese people often have increased levels of insulin and insulin-like growth factor-1 (IGF-1) in their blood (a condition known as hyperinsulinemia or insulin resistance), which may promote the development of certain tumors.
- Fat cells produce hormones, called adipokines, that may stimulate or inhibit cell growth. For example, leptin, which is more abundant in obese people, seems to promote cell proliferation, whereas adiponectin, which is less abundant in obese people, may have antiproliferative effects.
- Fat cells may also have direct and indirect effects on other tumor growth regulators, including mammalian target of rapamycin (mTOR) and AMP-activated protein kinase.

- Obese people often have chronic low-level, or "subacute," inflammation, which has been associated with increased cancer risk.

Other possible mechanisms include altered immune responses, effects on the nuclear factor kappa beta system, and oxidative stress.

What is known about the relationship between obesity and breast cancer?

Many studies have shown that overweight and obesity are associated with a modest increase in risk of postmenopausal breast cancer. This higher risk is seen mainly in women who have never used menopausal hormone therapy (MHT) and for tumors that express both estrogen and progesterone receptors.

Overweight and obesity have, by contrast, been found to be associated with a reduced risk of premenopausal breast cancer in some studies.

The relationship between obesity and breast cancer may be affected by the stage of life in which a woman gains weight and becomes obese. Epidemiologists are actively working to address this question. Weight gain during adult life, most often from about age 18 to between the ages of 50 and 60, has been consistently associated with risk of breast cancer after menopause.

The increased risk of postmenopausal breast cancer is thought to be due to increased levels of estrogen in obese women. After menopause, when the ovaries stop producing hormones, fat tissue becomes the most important source of estrogen. Because obese women have more fat tissue, their estrogen levels are higher, potentially leading to more rapid growth of estrogen-responsive breast tumors.

The relationship between obesity and breast cancer risk may also vary by race and ethnicity. There is limited evidence that the risk associated with overweight and obesity may be less among African American and Hispanic women than among white women.

What is known about the relationship between obesity and endometrial cancer?

Overweight and obesity have been consistently associated with endometrial cancer, which is cancer of the lining of the uterus. Obese and overweight women have two to four times the risk of developing this disease than women of a normal weight, regardless of menopausal status. Many studies have also found that the risk of endometrial cancer increases with increasing weight gain in adulthood, particularly among women who have never used MHT.

Although it has not yet been determined why obesity is a risk factor for endometrial cancer, some evidence points to a role for diabetes, possibly in combination with low levels of physical activity. High levels of estrogen produced by fat tissue are also likely to play a role.

What is known about the relationship between obesity and colorectal cancer?

Among men, a higher BMI is strongly associated with increased risk of colorectal cancer. The distribution of body fat appears to be an important factor, with abdominal obesity, which can be measured by waist circumference, showing the strongest association with colon cancer risk.

An association between BMI and waist circumference with colon cancer risk is also seen in women, but it is weaker. Use of MHT may modify the association in postmenopausal women.

A number of mechanisms have been proposed to account for the association of obesity with increased colon cancer risk. One hypothesis is that high levels of insulin or insulin-related growth factors in obese people may promote colon cancer development.

High BMI is also associated with rectal cancer risk, but the increase in risk is more modest.

What is known about the relationship between obesity and kidney cancer?

Obesity has been consistently associated with renal cell cancer, which is the most common form of kidney cancer, in both men and women. The mechanisms by which obesity may increase renal cell cancer risk are not well understood. High blood pressure is a known risk factor for renal cell cancer, but the relationship between obesity and kidney cancer is independent of blood pressure status. High levels of insulin may play a role in the development of the disease.

What is known about the relationship between obesity and esophageal cancer?

Overweight and obese people are about twice as likely as people of healthy weight to develop a type of esophageal cancer called esophageal adenocarcinoma. Most studies have observed no increased risk, or even a decline in risk, with obesity for the other major type of esophageal cancer, squamous cell cancer.

The mechanisms by which obesity may increase risk of esophageal adenocarcinoma are not well understood. However, overweight and obese people are more likely than people of normal weight to have a history of gastroesophageal reflux disease or Barrett esophagus, which are associated with an increased risk of esophageal adenocarcinoma. It is possible that obesity exacerbates the esophageal inflammation that is associated with these conditions.

What is known about the relationship between obesity and pancreatic cancer?

Many studies have reported a slight increase in risk of pancreatic cancer among overweight and obese individuals. Waist circumference may be a particularly important factor in the association of overweight and obesity with pancreatic cancer.

What is known about the relationship between obesity and thyroid cancer?

Increasing weight has been found to be associated with an increase in the risk of thyroid cancer. It is unclear what the mechanism might be.

What is known about the relationship between obesity and gallbladder cancer?

The risk of gallbladder cancer increases with increasing BMI. The increase in risk may be due to the higher frequency of gallstones, a strong risk factor for gallbladder cancer, in obese individuals.

What is known about the relationship between obesity and other cancers?

The relationship between obesity and prostate cancer has been studied extensively. The results of individual studies do not suggest a consistent association between obesity and prostate cancer. However, when the data from multiple studies are pooled, analyses show that obesity may be associated with a very slight increase in the risk of prostate cancer.

In addition, several studies have found that obese men have a higher risk of aggressive prostate cancer than men of healthy weight. Generally, risk of prostate cancer has been linked to levels of certain hormones and growth factors, especially IGF-1.

Some studies have shown a weak association between increasing BMI and risk of ovarian cancer, especially in premenopausal women, although other studies have not found an association. As with some other cancers, an association between ovarian cancer and obesity may reflect increased levels of estrogens.

Some evidence links obesity to liver cancer and to some types of lymphoma and leukemia, but additional studies are needed to confirm these associations.

Does avoiding weight gain or losing weight decrease the risk of cancer?

The most conclusive way to test whether avoiding weight gain or losing weight will decrease the risk of cancer is through a controlled clinical trial. A number of NIH-funded weight loss trials have demonstrated that people can lose weight and that losing weight reduces their risk of developing chronic diseases, such as diabetes, while improving their risk factors for cardiovascular disease.

However, previous trials and the results of an NCI workshop have demonstrated that it would not be feasible to conduct a weight loss trial of cancer prevention. The reason is that the effect of weight loss on the prevention of other chronic diseases would be demonstrated—and the trial consequently stopped so that the public could be informed of the benefits—before the effect on the prevention of cancer would become evident.

Therefore, most data about whether losing weight or avoiding weight gain prevents cancer come mainly from cohort and case-control studies. Data from these types of studies, called observational studies, can be difficult to interpret because people who lose weight or avoid weight gain may be different in other ways from people who do not, just as obese people may differ from lean people in other ways than BMI. That is, it is possible that these other differences explain their different cancer risk.

Nevertheless, many observational studies have shown that people who have a lower weight gain during adulthood have a lower risk of:

- Colon cancer
- Breast cancer (after menopause)
- Endometrial cancer

A more limited number of observational studies have examined the relationship between weight loss and cancer risk, and a few have found decreased risks of breast cancer and colon cancer among people who have lost weight. However, most of these studies have not been able to evaluate whether the weight loss was intentional or related to underlying health problems.

Stronger evidence comes from studies of patients who have undergone bariatric surgery to lose weight. Obese people who have bariatric surgery appear to have lower rates of obesity-related cancers than obese people who did not have bariatric surgery. It is important to note that whereas most lifestyle weight loss interventions result in weight losses of 7-10 percent of body weight, weight loss from bariatric surgery combined with lifestyle changes generally results in weight loss of 30 percent.

Chapter 6: Genetics

Scientists have made great advances in understanding important environmental causes of obesity as well as identifying several genes that might be implicated. Major efforts are now directed towards assessing the interactions of genes and environment in the obesity epidemic.

Obesity results when body fat accumulates over time as a result of a chronic energy imbalance (calories consumed exceed calories expended). Obesity is a major health hazard worldwide and is associated with several relatively common diseases such as diabetes, hypertension, heart disease, and some cancers.

The "Obesity Epidemic"–Can Genes Really Be Involved?

In recent decades, obesity has reached epidemic proportions in populations whose environments offer an abundance of calorie-rich foods and few opportunities for physical activity. Although changes in the genetic makeup of populations occur too slowly to be responsible for this rapid rise in obesity, genes do play a role in the development of obesity. Most likely, genes regulate how our bodies capture, store, and release energy from food. The origin of these genes, however, might not be recent.

How Might Genes Contribute to Obesity? A "Thrifty Genotype" Hypothesis

Any explanation of the obesity epidemic has to include both the role of genetics as well as that of the environment. A commonly quoted genetic explanation for the rapid rise in obesity is the mismatch between today's environment and "energy-thrifty genes" that multiplied in the past under different environmental conditions when food sources were rather unpredictable. In other words, according to the "thrifty genotype" hypothesis, the same genes that helped our ancestors survive occasional famines are now being challenged by environments in which food is plentiful year round.

What Other Ways Might Genes Influence Obesity?

It has been argued that the thrifty genotype is just part of a wider spectrum of ways in which genes can favor fat accumulation in a given environment. These ways include the drive to overeat (poor regulation of appetite and satiety); the tendency to be sedentary (physically inactive); a diminished ability to use dietary fats as fuel; and an enlarged, easily stimulated capacity to store body fat. Not all people living in industrialized countries with abundant food and reduced physical activity are or will become obese; nor will all obese people have the same body fat distribution or suffer the same health issues. This diversity occurs among groups of the same racial or ethnic background and even within families living in the same environment. The variation in how people respond to the same environmental conditions is an additional indication that genes play a role in the development of obesity. This is consistent with the theory that obesity results from genetic variation interacting with shifting environmental conditions.

What Do We Know about Specific Genes Associated with Obesity?

The indirect scientific evidence for a genetic basis for obesity comes from a variety of studies. Mostly, this evidence includes studies of resemblance and differences among family members, twins, and adoptees. Another source of evidence includes studies that have found some genes at higher frequencies among the obese (association studies). These investigations suggest that a sizable portion of the weight variation in adults is due to genetic factors. However, identifying these factors has been difficult.

How Can Public Health Genomics Help Reduce the Impact of Obesity in Populations?

Scientists have made great advances in understanding important environmental causes of obesity as well as identifying several of the many genes that might be implicated. Major efforts are now directed toward assessing the interactions of genes and environment in the obesity epidemic. The translation of these efforts into public health practice, from a genomic point of view, will take time.

How Can Family History Help?

Fortunately, there is a simple way for public health genomics to start reducing the effects of obesity in populations. It is through the use of family history. Family history reflects genetic susceptibility and environmental exposures shared by close relatives. Health care practitioners can routinely collect family health history to help identify people at high risk of obesity-related disorders such as diabetes, cardiovascular diseases, and some forms of cancer. Weight loss or prevention of excessive weight gains is especially important in this high-risk group. Any health promotion effort to reduce the adverse impact of obesity in populations may be more effective if it directs more intensive lifestyle interventions to high-risk groups (high-risk prevention strategy). However, such strategies should not detract from the population prevention strategy, which recommends that regardless of genetic susceptibility and environmental exposure, all people should follow a healthful diet and incorporate regular physical activity into their daily routine to help reduce the risk of obesity and its associated conditions.

Chapter 7: Child Obesity

Obesity means having too much body fat. It is different from being overweight, which means weighing too much. Both terms mean that a person's weight is greater than what's considered healthy for his or her height. Children grow at different rates, so it isn't always easy to know when a child is obese or overweight. Ask your health care provider to check whether your child's weight and height are in a healthy range.

If a weight-loss program is necessary, involve the whole family in healthy habits so your child doesn't feel singled out. Encourage healthy eating by

- Serving more fruits and vegetables
- Buying fewer soft drinks and high-fat, high-calorie snack foods
- Making sure your child eats breakfast every day
- Eating fast food less often
- Not using food as a reward

Physical activity is also very important. Kids need about 60 minutes each day. It does not have to happen all at once. Several short periods of activity during the day are just as good.

More than 35% of U.S. adults are obese, and more than 34% are overweight. Obesity affects 17% of all children and adolescents in the United States, which is three times the prevalence from just one generation ago. Nearly 32% of children and adolescents are either overweight or obese.

Helping Your Overweight Child

Is my child overweight?

Children grow at different rates at different times, so it is not always easy to tell if a child is overweight. If you think that your child is overweight, talk to your health care provider. He or she can tell you if your child's weight and height are in a healthy range.

How can I help my overweight child?

Involve the whole family in building healthy eating and physical activity habits. This benefits everyone and does not single out the child who is overweight.

Do not put your child on a weight-loss diet unless your health care provider tells you to. If children do not eat enough, they may not grow and learn as well as they should.

Be supportive

- Tell your child that he or she is loved, special, and important. Children's feelings about themselves are often based on how they think their parents feel about them.
- Accept your child at any weight. Children are more likely to accept and feel good about themselves when their parents accept them.
- Listen to your child's concerns about his or her weight. Overweight children probably know better than anyone else that they have a weight problem. They need support, understanding, and encouragement from parents.

Encourage healthy eating habits

- Buy and serve more fruits and vegetables (fresh, frozen, canned, or dried). Let your child choose them at the store.
- Buy fewer soft drinks and high-fat or high-calorie snack foods like chips, cookies, and candy. These snacks may be OK once in a while, but always keep healthy snack foods on hand. Offer the healthy snacks more often at snack times.
- Make sure your child eats breakfast every day. Breakfast may provide your child with the energy he or she needs to listen and learn in school. Skipping breakfast can leave your child hungry, tired, and looking for less healthy foods later in the day.
- Eat fast food less often. When you do visit a fast food restaurant, encourage your family to choose the healthier options, such as salads with low-fat dressing or small sandwiches without cheese or mayonnaise.
- Offer your child water or low-fat milk more often than fruit juice. Low-fat milk and milk products are important for your child's development. One hundred percent fruit juice is a healthy choice but is high in calories.
- Limit the amount of saturated and trans fats in your family's diet. Instead, obtain most of your fats from sources such as fish, vegetable oils, nuts, and seeds.
- Plan healthy meals and eat together as a family. Eating together at meal times helps children learn to enjoy a variety of foods.

- Do not get discouraged if your child will not eat a new food the first time it is served. Some kids will need to have a new food served to them 10 times or more before they will eat it.
- Try not to use food as a reward when encouraging kids to eat. Promising dessert to a child for eating vegetables, for example, sends the message that vegetables are less valuable than dessert. Kids learn to dislike foods they think are less valuable.
- Start with small servings and let your child ask for more if he or she is still hungry. It is up to you to provide your child with healthy meals and snacks, but your child should be allowed to choose how much food he or she will eat.
- Be aware that some high-fat or high-sugar foods and beverages may be strongly marketed to kids. Usually these products are associated with cartoon characters, offer free toys, and come in bright packages. Talk with your child about the importance of fruits, vegetables, whole grains, and other healthy foods— even if these foods are not often advertised on TV or in stores.
- Healthy Snack Ideas-Your child might enjoy trying the following foods:

  o Fresh fruit.
  o Fruit canned in juice or light syrup.
  o Small amounts of dried fruits, such as raisins, apple rings, or apricots.
  o Fresh vegetables, such as baby carrots, cucumber, zucchini, or tomatoes.

- Low-sugar, whole-grain cereal with low-fat milk.
- Foods that are small, round, sticky, or hard to chew, such as raisins, whole grapes, hard vegetables, hard chunks of cheese, nuts, seeds, and popcorn, can cause choking in children under age 4. You can still prepare some of these foods for young children, for example, by cutting grapes into small pieces and cooking and cutting up vegetables. Always watch your toddler during meals and snacks.

Encourage daily physical activity

Like adults, kids need daily physical activity. Here are some ways to help your child move every day:

- Set a good example. If your child sees that you are physically active and that you have fun doing it, he or she is more likely to be active throughout life.
- Encourage your child to join a sports team or class, such as soccer, dance, basketball, or gymnastics at school or at your local community or recreation center.
- Be sensitive to your child's needs. If your child feels uncomfortable participating in activities like sports, help him or her find physical activities that are fun and not embarrassing, such as playing tag with friends or siblings, jumping rope, or dancing to his or her favorite music.
- Be active together as a family. Assign active chores such as making the beds, washing the car, or

vacuuming. Plan active outings such as a trip to the zoo, a family bike ride, or a walk through a local park.

A pre-adolescent child's body is not ready for adult-style physical activity. Do not encourage your child to participate in activities such as long jogs, using an exercise bike or treadmill, or lifting heavy weights. FUN physical activities that kids choose to do on their own are often best.

Kids need about 60 minutes of physical activity a day, but this does not have to happen all at once. Several short 10- or even 5-minute periods of activity throughout the day are just as good. If your children are not used to being active, encourage them to start with what they can do and build up to 60 minutes a day.

FUN Physical Activity Ideas

- Riding a bike
- Climbing on a jungle gym
- Jumping rope
- Playing hopscotch
- Bouncing a ball
- Dancing
- Playing catch

Discourage inactive pastimes

- Set limits on the amount of time your family spends watching TV, playing video games, and being on the computer.

- Help your child find FUN things to do besides watching TV, like acting out favorite books or stories, or doing a family art project. Your child may find that creative play is more interesting than TV.
- Encourage your child to get up and move during commercials and discourage snacking when the TV is on.

Be a positive role model

Children are good learners and they often mimic what they see. Choose healthy foods and active pastimes for yourself. Your children will learn to follow healthy habits that last a lifetime.

Resources

- BAM! Body and Mind answers kids' questions about health, including physical activity and nutrition. It also offers a "Teacher's Corner" for educators. http://www.bam.gov
- ChooseMyPlate offers information about making healthier food choices and being active. http://www.choosemyplate.gov
- Fruits and Veggies—More Matters is a joint initiative from the Centers for Disease Control and Prevention and the Produce for Better Health Foundation to encourage Americans to eat more fruits and vegetables. The initiative's website offers nutritional information, recipes, and tips. http://www.fruitsandveggiesmatter.gov
- KidsHealth offers nutrition and fitness information for kids. http://www.kidshealth.org

- Kidnetic provides tips on healthy eating and physical activity for kids and parents. http://www.kidnetic.com
- National Diabetes Education Program provides information about diabetes and children to parents and health care professionals. http://www.ndep.nih.gov/diabetes/youth/youth.htm
- Verb is a website that encourages kids to be physically active. http://www.cdc.gov
- WeCan! Ways to Enhance Children's Activity and Nutrition is a national program designed for families and communities to help children maintain a healthy weight. http://www.nhlbi.nih.gov/health/public/heart/obesity/wecan/index.htm

Chapter 8: Women's Obesity

How many women in the United States are overweight or obese?

Over 60 percent of U.S. adult women are overweight, according to 2007 estimates from the National Center for Health Statistics of the Center for Disease Control and Prevention. Just over one-third of overweight adult women are obese

How do I know if I'm overweight or obese?

Find out your body mass index (BMI). BMI is a measure of body fat based on height and weight. People with a BMI of 25 to 29.9 are considered overweight. People with a BMI of 30 or more are considered obese.

What causes someone to become overweight or obese?

You can become overweight or obese when you eat more calories (KAL-oh-rees) than you use. A calorie is a unit of energy in the food you eat. Your body needs this energy to function and to be active. But if you take in more energy than your body uses, you will gain weight.

Many factors can play a role in becoming overweight or obese. These factors include:

- Behaviors, such as eating too many calories or not getting enough physical activity
- Environment and culture
- Genes

Overweight and obesity problems keep getting worse in the United States. Some cultural reasons for this include:

- Bigger portion sizes
- Little time to exercise or cook healthy meals
- Using cars to get places instead of walking

What are the health effects of being overweight or obese?

Being overweight or obese can increase your risk of:

- Heart disease
- Stroke
- Type 2 diabetes
- High blood pressure
- Breathing problems
- Arthritis
- Gallbladder disease
- Some kinds of cancer

But excess body weight isn't the only health risk. The places where you store your body fat also affect your health. Women with a "pear" shape tend to store fat in their hips and buttocks. Women with an "apple" shape store fat around their waists. If your waist is more than 35 inches, you may have a higher risk of weight-related health problems.

What is the best way for me to lose weight?

The best way to lose weight is to use more calories than you take in. You can do this by following a healthy eating plan and being more active. Before you start a weight-loss program, talk to your doctor.

Safe weight-loss programs that work well:

- Set a goal of slow and steady weight loss — 1 to 2 pounds per week
- Offer low-calorie eating plans with a wide range of healthy foods
- Encourage you to be more physically active
- Teach you about healthy eating and physical activity
- Adapt to your likes and dislikes and cultural background
- Help you keep weight off after you lose it

How can I make healthier food choices?

The U.S. Department of Health and Human Services (HHS) and Department of Agriculture (USDA) offer tips for healthy eating in Dietary Guidelines for All Americans.

- Focus on fruits. Eat a variety of fruits — fresh, frozen, canned, or dried — rather than fruit juice for most of your fruit choices. For a 2,000-calorie diet, you will need 2 cups of fruit each day. An example of 2 cups is 1 small banana, 1 large orange, and 1/4 cup of dried apricots or peaches.
- Vary your veggies. Eat more:
  - dark green veggies, such as broccoli, kale, and other dark leafy greens
  - orange veggies, such as carrots, sweet potatoes, pumpkin, and winter squash
  - beans and peas, such as pinto beans, kidney beans, black beans, garbanzo beans, split peas, and lentils

- Get your calcium-rich foods. Each day, drink 3 cups of low-fat or fat-free milk. Or, you can get an equivalent amount of low-fat yogurt and/or low-fat cheese each day. 1.5 ounces of cheese equals 1 cup of milk. If you don't or can't consume milk, choose lactose-free milk products and/or calcium-fortified foods and drinks.
- Make half your grains whole. Eat at least 3 ounces of whole-grain cereals, breads, crackers, rice, or pasta each day. One ounce is about 1 slice of bread, 1 cup of breakfast cereal, or 1/2 cup of cooked rice or pasta. Look to see that grains such as wheat, rice, oats, or corn are referred to as "whole" in the list of ingredients.
- Go lean with protein. Choose lean meats and poultry. Bake it, broil it, or grill it. Vary your protein choices with more fish, beans, peas, nuts, and seeds.
- Limit saturated fats. Get less than 10 percent of your calories from saturated fatty acids. Most fats should come from sources of polyunsaturated and monounsaturated fatty acids, such as fish, nuts, and vegetable oils. When choosing and preparing meat, poultry, dry beans, and milk or milk products, make choices that are lean, low-fat, or fat-free.
- Limit salt. Get less than 2,300 mg of sodium (about 1 teaspoon of salt) each day.

How can physical activity help?

The new 2008 Physical Activity Guidelines for Americans state that an active lifestyle can lower your risk of early death from a variety of causes. There is strong evidence that regular physical activity can also lower your risk of:

- Heart disease
- Stroke
- High blood pressure
- Unhealthy cholesterol levels
- Type 2 diabetes
- Metabolic syndrome
- Colon cancer
- Breast cancer
- Falls
- Depression

Regular activity can help prevent unhealthy weight gain and also help with weight loss, when combined with lower calorie intake. If you are overweight or obese, losing weight can lower your risk for many diseases. Being overweight or obese increases your risk of heart disease, high blood pressure, stroke, type 2 diabetes, breathing problems, osteoarthritis, gallbladder disease, sleep apnea (breathing problems while sleeping), and some cancers.

Regular physical activity can also improve your cardiorespiratory (heart, lungs, and blood vessels) and muscular fitness. For older adults, activity can improve mental function.

Physical activity may also help:

- Improve functional health for older adults
- Reduce waistline size
- Lower risk of hip fracture

- Lower risk of lung cancer
- Lower risk of endometrial cancer
- Maintain weight after weight loss
- Increase bone density
- Improve sleep quality

Health benefits are gained by doing one of the following each week:

- 2 hours and 30 minutes of moderate-intensity aerobic physical activity
- 1 hour and 15 minutes of vigorous-intensity aerobic physical activity
- A combination of moderate and vigorous-intensity aerobic physical activity
- Muscle-strengthening activities on 2 or more days

This physical activity should be in addition to your routine activities of daily living, such as cleaning or spending a few minutes walking from the parking lot to your office.

If you want to lose a substantial (more than 5 percent of body weight) amount of weight, you need a high amount of physical activity unless you also lower calorie intake. This is also the case if you are trying to keep the weight off. Many people need to do more than 300 minutes of moderate-intensity activity a week to meet weight-control goals.

How you can increase your physical activity

If you normally...	Try this instead!
Park as close as possible to the store	Park farther away

Let the dog out back	Take the dog for a walk
Take the elevator	Take the stairs
Have lunch delivered	Walk to pick up lunch
Relax while the kids play	Get involved in their activity

What medicines are approved for long-term treatment of obesity?

The Food and Drug Administration has approved two medicines for long-term treatment of obesity:

- Sibutramine (si-BYOO-tra-meen) suppresses your appetite.
- Orlistat (OR-li-stat) keeps your body from absorbing fat from the food you eat.

These medicines are for people who:

- Have a BMI of 30 or higher
- Have a BMI of 27 or higher and weight-related health problems or health risks

If you take these medicines, you will need to follow a healthy eating and physical activity plan at the same time.

Before taking these medicines, talk with your doctor about the benefits and the side effects.

- Sibutramine can raise your blood pressure and heart rate. You should not take this medicine if you have a history of high blood pressure, heart problems, or strokes. Other side effects include dry mouth, headache, constipation, anxiety, and trouble sleeping.
- Orlistat may cause diarrhea, cramping, gas, and leakage of oily stool. Eating a low-fat diet can help prevent these side effects. This medicine may also prevent your body from absorbing some vitamins. Talk with your doctor about whether you should take a vitamin supplement.

What surgical options are used to treat obesity?

Weight loss surgeries — also called bariatric (bair-ee-AT-rik) surgeries — can help treat obesity. You should only consider surgical treatment for weight loss if you:

- Have a BMI of 40 or higher
- Have a BMI of 35 or higher and weight-related health problems
- Have not had success with other weight-loss methods

Common types of weight loss surgeries are:

- Roux-en-Y (ROO-en-WEYE) gastric bypass. The surgeon uses surgical staples to create a small stomach pouch. This limits the amount of food you can eat. The pouch is attached to the middle part of the small intestine. Food bypasses the upper part of the small intestine and stomach, reducing the amount of calories and nutrients your body absorbs.

- Laparoscopic (LAP-uh-ruh-SKAWP-ik) gastric banding. A band is placed around the upper stomach to create a small pouch and narrow passage into the rest of the stomach. This limits the amount of food you can eat. The size of the band can be adjusted. A surgeon can remove the band if needed.
- Biliopancreatic (bil-ee-oh-pan-kree-at-ik) diversion (BPD) or BPD with duodenal (doo-AW-duh-nul) switch (BPD/DS). In BPD, a large part of the stomach is removed, leaving a small pouch. The pouch is connected to the last part of the small intestine, bypassing other parts of the small intestine. In BPD/DS, less of the stomach and small intestine are removed. This surgery reduces the amount of food you can eat and the amount of calories and nutrients your body absorbs from food. This surgery is used less often than other types of surgery because of the high risk of malnutrition.

If you are thinking about weight-loss surgery, talk with your doctor about changes you will need to make after the surgery. You will need to:

- Follow your doctor's directions as you heal
- Make lasting changes in the way you eat
- Follow a healthy eating plan and be physically active
- Take vitamins and minerals if needed

You should also talk to your doctor about risks and side effects of weight loss surgery. Side effects may include:

- Infection

- Leaking from staples
- Hernia
- Blood clots in the leg veins that travel to your lungs (pulmonary embolism)
- Dumping syndrome, in which food moves from your stomach to your intestines too quickly
- Not getting enough vitamins and minerals from food

Is liposuction a treatment for obesity?

Liposuction (LY-poh-suhk-shuhn) is not a treatment for obesity. In this procedure, a surgeon removes fat from under the skin. Liposuction can be used to reshape parts of your body. But this surgery does not promise lasting weight loss.

www.MedicalCenter.com

www.ingramcontent.com/pod-product-compliance
Lightning Source LLC
Chambersburg PA
CBHW070555290526
45790CB00002B/695